The Beauty Buzz

NO MORE BEAUTY B.S.!

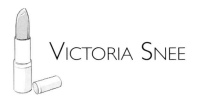

VICTORIA SNEE

The Beauty Buzz
No More Beauty B.S.

Brown Books Publishing Group
16200 North Dallas Parkway, Suite 170
Dallas, Texas 75248
www.brownbooks.com
(972) 381-0009

A New Era in Publishing™

ISBN 978-1-934812-87-7
Library of Congress Control Number 2010937788

Printed in the United States of America.
10 9 8 7 6 5 4 3 2 1

Author photos by David Woo
Illustrations by Ralph Voltz

For more information about Victoria Snee and *The Beauty Buzz*, please visit www.beautybuzzbook.com.

For my loving Mom-Mom, whose beauty I miss every day.

TABLE OF CONTENTS

NO MORE BEAUTY B.S.!
Introduction

Are you as tired of the Beauty B.S. as I am? You know what it's like. You walk into a department store and are attacked by a bored salesperson, who doesn't know you, but who is just dying to give you a make-over and sell you every product under the sun. Then, it's like you've slipped into a cosmetic coma. They're going on about plumping and lengthening and moisturizing, but your mind has gone blank. The next thing you know, a stranger, whose face is covered in mounds of make-up, is looking back at you from the mirror and your credit card has just been charged $400 for things like bright pink lipstick and colored mascara that only your teenage niece would wear. If this hasn't happened to you, consider yourself lucky. Lord knows it's happened to me! That's why I'm here to help wake you up from the beauty blackout you've been in for years.

I am not a make-up artist, and I do not work for a cosmetics line—but I am a full-fledged beauty junkie. I love beauty products. The cosmetics department in any major store is my mecca, and I never know where to look first! What is catching my eye? Is it the long line of lip glosses in pretty tubes or sleek, slender cases? Or maybe the eye shadow palettes bursting with colors like rich brown amaretto, emerald green, perfect plum, or ocean blue? Who can resist the tempting jars of moisturizers, hand creams, and eye serums? I immediately want to try them all. When I'm having a bad day or I'm out shopping and nothing seems to fit, the cosmetics counter is where I always end up. Make-up always seems to come in my size (thank goodness!), and a brand new tube of lipstick can instantly put a smile on my face.

I'm telling you all of this because, when it comes to products, I have tested and tried dozens and dozens of them. I know what works and what doesn't. I spent ten years of my career working as a fashion/lifestyle/entertainment reporter on television, which means I've interviewed countless Hollywood stars and had the opportunity to meet and talk to their make-up artists, too. I loved chatting with those cosmetics specialists to the stars about their tips, tricks, and little secrets to play up everyone's best features while hiding the common beauty flaws that make many of us cringe when we look in the mirror. (This is where I first learned that lining the inner rims of your eyes with white eyeliner pencil could make you look awake when you are actually sleep-deprived.)

The make-up artists weren't the only ones who liked to share their wisdom about eyeliner pencils and powder blushes—the celebrities themselves were always gracious in sharing their favorite beauty products and the skills they learned in the business. I've also interviewed several of the biggest names in the beauty industry, from Bobbi Brown to Laura Mercier to Aerin Lauder. I learned so much from these beautiful women, and now I get to share it all with you.

Besides my work in television, I've also worked in radio for several years, co-hosting a morning show in

Dallas. In 2007, I started my weekly Beauty Buzz segment, where I take beauty questions from listeners who need help with everything from applying self-tanners to picking out the right brand of mascara to figuring out what skincare products to use. You will see some of their questions at the beginning of each chapter of *The Beauty Buzz*.

Each chapter of the book addresses what I like to call the beauty basics—choosing the right skincare products, foundation color, eye shadow shade, lipstick color, cheek color, etc. I will give you tips and tricks on how to choose the proper products, how to apply them, and which items I have found work the best. I will list products that I think are worth your beauty bucks and some that I think you can save on. You will know which ones to save on by the clearly marked Beauty Saver Symbol ($). I also like to end each chapter with a celebrity story called "Star Style." These anecdotes come from the countless celebrity interviews I've done over the years. I was always asking actresses beauty questions, even when I was really there to talk to them about their latest horror film or romantic comedy!

This books cuts to the chase. There's No Beauty B.S. here—I'm giving you the Straight Buzz. I've done all the research for you and asked all the questions. The tips in this book work, plain and simple. I want this book to be a resource for you for everything from basic skincare to the perfect lip liner. When you go beauty shopping, I want you to slip *The Beauty Buzz* into your purse and take it with you. So, let's cut the cosmetics crap and get gorgeous together!

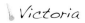

Victoria

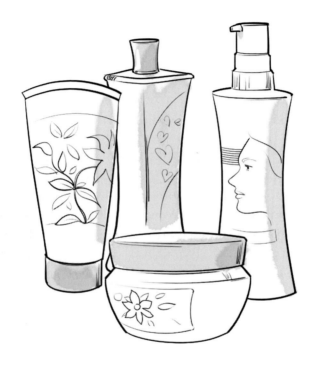

Question from Jennifer

Can you help me with figuring out the order in which I should do my facial cleansing routine morning and night? Example: make-up remover, then toner, then exfoliator, then moisturizer and mask (once a week)?

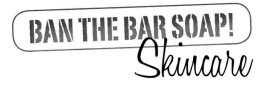

BAN THE BAR SOAP!
Skincare

Here's the deal, ladies. I don't care how much you spend on fancy foundation, expensive eye shadow, or luxurious lip gloss. There is *nothing* more important than skincare. If your skin isn't in prime condition, none of the products you buy are going to look good or help you realize your full beauty potential. Your skin HAS to be in tip-top shape, or no amount of make-up is going to be able to mask what's really going on. It's all about the state of your skin. You've heard of the State of the Union address, right? Well, consider this section your State of the Skin address. Now that we live in an HD world, it's officially on!

I can't say it enough: Your make-up will never look great until your skin looks great. That's because make-up is not meant to mask your imperfections. It's meant to enhance your natural beauty. Once you get your skin looking its very best, you can focus on using make-up to bring out your most beautiful features. This is so important, and it's easy to achieve, too—there are certain no-hassle steps you can take in your daily life to avoid basic beauty offenses that keep you from looking your best! PLEASE don't tell me that you still sleep in your make-up, use a bar soap as a cleanser, or don't regularly use moisturizer and eye cream. If you've answered "yes" to any of these, I am so glad you bought this book! We are going to change those bad habits NOW!

If you're thinking to yourself, this is going to cost me a small fortune, think again. Great skincare doesn't have to cost a lot of money. There are amazing products you can find in the drugstore that work just as well as some of those fancy products you see in the department stores. There are some products worth the splurge and some you can definitely save your beauty bucks on. Don't worry—I'll let you know what they are at the end of this chapter.

READY, SET, PREP!

Your clean, fresh face is your canvas, so before you grab your blush brush and mascara wand, take some time to do some basic prep work.

First, start off by making sure that you have these skincare products in your beauty wardrobe (yes, it is a wardrobe!): cleanser, toner, eye cream, serum, moisturizer, and make-up remover.

To answer Jennifer's question from page 4, this is the proper order to apply the skincare products I've just listed (and I've explained each step in great detail on the following page):

DAY	NIGHT
Cleanser	Make-Up Remover
Toner	Cleanser
Eye Cream	Toner
Serum	Eye Cream
Moisturizer	Moisturizer
Make-Up Primer	
Sunscreen	

Cleanser

Are you using bar soap on your face? Are you kidding me!? Stop that right now! Bar soap is much too drying, and you really need to use something less harsh on your skin. One of my favorite products that works especially well for sensitive skin is Cetaphil. You can buy it at the drugstore, and even dermatologists recommend it. Some other affordable cleansers I love are Olay's Moisture Balancing Foaming Face Wash and Olay's Age Defying Daily Renewal Cleanser. I also love Renée Rouleau's Luxe Mint Cleansing Gel.

Remember, your face should never feel tight or dry after cleansing. If it does, switch products immediately.

Toner

A word about toners. Some people skip this step in their skincare routine, but I really love using a good toner right after I cleanse. It helps tighten the skin and stimulates collagen production. (This is important, because we lose collagen as we age.) A toner makes my skin feel fresh and removes any trace of make-up that I might have missed. If you do use a toner, make sure it's alcohol-free. You don't want it to dry out your skin.

Eye Cream

The eyes will always have it. To keep your peepers looking perfect, apply an eye cream twice daily (morning and night). Be sure and use your ring finger, since it applies the least amount of pressure to that delicate skin area. I think it's so important to truly pamper the area around your eyes. Your eyes are the window to your soul, after all, but they're also one of the first areas to show those fine lines and wrinkles—and you want those windows to look young! Splurge on a really good eye cream. It's worth every cent.

Serum

A serum is a product that sinks within your skin and carries active ingredients beneath the skin's surface. Because a serum is made of smaller molecules, it can actually penetrate all three layers of skin and work from the inside out! This means a serum can help with common problems like fine lines and wrinkles. Get one and use it every day. It will drastically improve your skin's look and texture.

Moisturizer

It still amazes me how many women I meet who say they don't use a daily moisturizer. Why not? It is one of the best and easiest things you can do for your skin. Fine lines will look more pronounced when the skin is dry and dehydrated, but a moisturizer can help restore that hydration back into the skin.

I like to use a light moisturizer for day and a heavy one at night. Our skin repairs itself while we sleep, so take advantage of your skin's natural cycle by using a more intense cream at night for maximum benefits.

Many moisturizers now come with an SPF. This is great, but only if it is at least an SPF 30. If not, you will have to use a separate sunscreen, which I will talk about coming up.

Even people with oily skin should use a moisturizer. When our skin is oily, we tend to want to dry the skin out, but that can actually make matters even worse. Your skin may start producing even more oil in order to compensate for the moisture you're taking away. In short, don't confuse oil with hydration. Your natural oil doesn't have the healing, restorative properties a moisturizer does.

Finally, don't neglect your neck! Nothing gives away your age faster. When you apply moisturizer, make sure to apply it there as well. You want that skin looking great, too! Many cosmetic lines make a separate neck cream, but if you can't afford the splurge, a regular moisturizer is better than nothing.

Make-Up Primer

Have you ever left the house, looked in the mirror a couple of hours later, and noticed half of your make-up is gone? It's like it evaporates or something! If you aren't using a make-up primer, BUY ONE! Primers help create a smooth, even canvas for applying your make-up. Think of yourself as an artist. You would never start painting on a bumpy, unsmooth surface, would you? No way! You would want a nice, clean canvas to work on—and it's the same for your face. A primer will fill in lines and pores so make-up won't settle in those areas. It acts as a barrier between your skin and your foundation. When you apply your primer, make sure to put it on right after your moisturizer and before your foundation. Laura Mercier and NARS both make great make-up primers.

Sunscreen

Are you still tanning your face? Are you nuts!? You are WAY too smart for that. The next thing you know, you are going to tell me that you are still smoking and lying like a corpse in tanning beds! Sun damage can add years to your face, not to mention the risk of cancer. I shouldn't have to tell you to use a daily sunscreen, but if you need me to, I will. USE A DAILY SUNSCREEN, and make sure it has an SPF of at least 30. Just like with a moisturizer, use it on your neck, too. It's the first part of the body that will show your age, so make sure you are protecting that delicate skin as well.

Taking It Off

When it comes to taking make-up off, I really like to do a thorough job. I use a couple of products to help me before I even reach for my cleanser. I like to use toning cloths or soft cotton circles or squares to remove my eye make-up. I have eyelash extensions (which I will talk about later in the book), so I need to use an oil-free remover. I really like Lancôme's Effacil eye make-up remover.

I also like to use a cleansing oil to remove foundation and concealer. Shu Uemura makes a great line of cleansing oils (Madonna loves this line of make-up). If you don't want to use an oil, Lancôme makes a cleansing water called Eau Fraîche Douceur that is great. MAC cosmetics also sells make-up remover wipes that are gentle on the skin and still get the job done.

Finally, if you are still sleeping in your make-up, STOP! There is nothing worse for your pores than sleeping in your make-up, and it makes a mess on your pillow! I know you're tired at the end of the day, but give your skin five minutes and take that make-up OFF. Your skin will thank you a few years down the road!

RENEW AND REFRESH: OTHER TIPS TO IMPROVE YOUR SKIN

I always get questions about ways to shrink pores. I have good news and some bad news. You can't shrink them, but you CAN minimize their appearance. In addition to taking off your make-up before you go to bed, make sure that you exfoliate at least twice a week to help remove dirt and bacteria, which can enlarge pore size. One of my favorite exfoliators is Renée Rouleau's Mint Buffing Beads.

Don't forget to exfoliate your neck, too! There is a two-step product by Philosophy called The Micro-delivery Peel. It will get rid of those dead skin cells, leaving skin feeling refreshed and renewed.

Make Sunday night your night to do something extra special for your skin. Sunday night is my own mini-facial night. I cleanse and tone my skin, then follow up with an exfoliator and apply a facial mask.

If you have dry to normal skin, look for a mask that is hydrating. For oily skin, a clay mask is a smart choice. I recommend you pick one night a week when you can give your skin some extra pampering. It deserves your time and attention.

Finally, if you can swing it financially, getting a professional facial every four to six weeks is ideal. But it can be pricey, and let's face it, we all have expensive shoes to buy! So, make a goal that you will at least try to get a professional facial every few months. You can keep up the results yourself if you are diligent about your at-home routine.

Treat Circles and Puffiness

Who doesn't love a late night out with the ladies? I've certainly had my share. We all have late nights, and yes, they often involve adult beverages. As we all painfully know, your skin will usually look a little less than gorgeous the next morning. Alcohol can quickly dehydrate the skin, and when you combine that with inadequate sleep, you'll definitely be looking less than festive. Try using products that contain a bit of caffeine to help minimize puffiness—when applied to the skin in certain creams and moisturizers, it can increase circulation and blood flow in areas where you need a beauty boost. I like Kiehl's Facial Fuel Eye De-Puffer and its Brightening Botanical Hydrating Mask. Origins' GinZing eye cream is great and also contains caffeine to help minimize puffiness.

So many women ask me about ways to treat dark circles. Even if you weren't sipping on a cocktail late into the night, lack of sleep alone can still leave you with those telltale tired rings. We all know we're supposed to get seven to eight hours of sleep a night, but come on! Seriously, who gets that much sleep these days!? With all the Facebooking and Tweeting we all do, it's a wonder we get any sleep at all! If you don't want dark circles, there's an easy solution: try to catch some more ZZZs. But dark circles can also be caused by a variety of other things, including genetics and age. The skin under the eye is super thin, which makes blood vessels more visible, and as you age the skin becomes even thinner, increasing the discoloration. In addition to trying to get more sleep, choose products that contain vitamin C, which can help fight those dark rings by minimizing melanin and adding volume to the skin. If all else fails, a great concealer will always be your best friend. I have what I consider a miracle concealer, and I will share it with you in a few chapters.

Banish Blemishes

We all HATE this topic, but blemishes are, unfortunately, a part of life. And they always seem to pop up, literally, at the worst times—just before a big party, date, business presentation, etc. Gross! Look for products that contain salicylic acid to dry them up. Some products I have used in the past that really work include Sonya Dakar's Drying Potion and Renée Rouleau's Anti-Cyst Treatment, as well as Night Time Spot Lotion.

You might not have considered it before, but another reason some break-outs happen? You're using make-up brushes that are dirty. NASTY! You need to clean your make-up brushes every week if possible. If not, don't go longer than two or three weeks. Think about it—you're putting that brush on your face every day, and it's exposed to all kinds of bacteria from your skin and from being left out in the elements. You need to clean them!

You don't need to buy any fancy make-up brush cleansers, although lots of cosmetics lines sell them. Just grab a bottle of Johnson's Baby Shampoo the next time you're at the drugstore. Put some in the palm of your hand along with some lukewarm water, take your brush, and swirl it around in the palm of your hand. Rinse the brush off and let it air dry on a towel for a few hours, and you're good to go.

 # HOW TO SPEND YOUR BEAUTY BUCKS—MY FAVORITE SKINCARE PRODUCTS

Cleansers

$ Cetaphil
Dermalogica Tri-Active Cleanse
$ Olay Moisture Balancing Foaming Face Wash
$ Olay Age Defying Daily Renewal Cleanser
Renée Rouleau Luxe Mint Cleansing Gel

Toners

Euoko Marine Vitamin Fluid
Lancôme Tonique Confort
Renée Rouleau Revitalizing Ginseng Toner

Eye Creams

Euoko Eye Contour Nanolift
Kiehl's Creamy Eye Treatment with Avocado
Kiehl's Facial Fuel Eye De-Puffer
La Mer The Eye Balm
Origins GinZing Eye Cream
RéVive Eye Renewal Cream
3LAB WW Eye Cream

Serums

Kate Sommerville Deep Tissue Repair
Kate Sommerville Quench
Kiehl's Midnight Recovery Concentrate
La Mer The Regenerating Serum
3LAB "h" Serum

Moisturizers

Dermalogica Skin Smoothing Cream
$ Olay Regenerist Micro-sculpting Cream
Philosophy Miracle Worker
3LAB Hydra Day SPF 20
3LAB "M" Cream

Make-Up Primers

Clé de Peau Smoothing Base for Lines or Pores
Laura Mercier Foundation Primer Hydrating
NARS Make-Up Primer
Smashbox Photo Finish Foundation Primer

Eye Make-Up Removers

Chanel Démaquillant Yeux Intense
Lancôme Bi-Facil Eye Make-Up Remover
Lancôme Effacil Eye Make-Up Remover

Make-Up Removers

Dermalogica Precleanse
Lancôme Eau Fraîche Douceur Cleansing Water
MAC Wipes
Shu Uemura Cleansing Oil

Exfoliants

Dermalogica Daily Microfoliant
Kate Sommerville ExfoliKate Intensive Exfoliating
  Treatment
Philosophy The Microdelivery Peel
Renée Rouleau Mint Buffing Beads
Renée Rouleau Triple Berry Smoothing Peel

Facial Masks

Euoko Extreme Cellular Nutrition Masque
Kiehl's Brightening Botanical Hydrating Mask
Lancôme Absolue Premium BX
NARS Aqua Gel Hydrator
3LAB Perfect Mask

Blemish Control

Renée Rouleau Anti-Cyst Treatment
Renée Rouleau Night Time Spot Lotion
Sonya Dakar Drying Potion

Sunscreens

Clinique Face Cream SPF 50
Renée Rouleau Daily Protection SPF 30
3LAB Perfect Sunscreen SPF 55

Star Style

Friends star Courteney Cox is one of the nicest actresses I've ever met. I interviewed her for the film *Scream 3* several years ago, and the minute I walked in the room to sit down and talk with her, she immediately gave me a big compliment on my skin. She told me how beautiful my skin was and asked me what products I was using. At the time, I was using La Mer. She said she had also used La Mer before and really liked it, too. It was just amazing to me that one of the biggest stars in television (she was still acting on *Friends* at the time) would want to make some beauty small talk with a complete stranger. She is a great, down-to-earth lady!

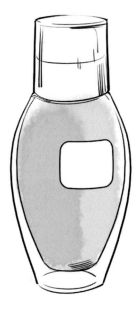

Question from Stephanie

I don't really like foundation and usually just use some powder on my face. But I feel like I do want a bit more coverage. Do you have any suggestions for a product that can give some coverage but won't look and feel too heavy?

NO MORE SCARY MASK FACE!
Foundation and Concealer

Now that we've finally tossed that bar soap out and focused on getting the flawless face we all want, it's time to start thinking about make-up application. If you still think you look great without make-up and you're over the age of thirty, you need to wake up and smell the foundation. When you get to a certain age, you need to wear make-up. Not even supermodels look good without it. Get real and get with the make-up program!

When you find the right shade of foundation and concealer for you, it can do wonders. Your skin will look smoother, and it creates a good canvas for applying blush and powder. There can be problems, though, when you wear a foundation shade that is wrong for you: It can end up looking like you're wearing a mask. NO SCARY MASK FACE! This is NOT a good look! You know what I'm talking about—the color of the face is four shades darker than the neck. You look like a giant orange pumpkin head. I don't even like Halloween in October, much less all year long! Here are some of my best tips on getting the right shade of foundation and concealer and making it work for you.

PICKING THE PERFECT FOUNDATION SHADE

There are many cosmetic items that you can save on, but when it comes to foundation and concealer, I think it's important to spend a little more on good quality products. These two items make such a big difference on your face. You can have on the coolest lip and eye color, but if your face looks orange from a bad foundation match or if your eyes have dark circles around them that aren't being covered up properly, no one will

Straight Buzz

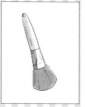

When I was in my twenties, I often used a powder foundation. MAC cosmetics makes one called Studio Fix that is wildly popular. But I have noticed that as I've gotten older, powder foundations are too dry for my skin. If you do like a powder foundation, by all means, use it. But remember, as we age, our skin does get drier, and powder can settle into fine lines. That's why I like to recommend a liquid foundation for more mature skin—it smoothes over and diminishes the look of fine lines, rather than emphasizing them.

see anything else. And there are so many different types of foundations to choose from—some offer full coverage, while others are more sheer, and there are also tinted moisturizers that are great to use in the summer when full foundations feel too heavy.

It's hard to tell if a foundation is right for you when you can't test it on your skin. That's why I don't buy these particular products in the drugstore. I usually recommend that women go to a cosmetics counter and get color-matched, meaning you find the shade that best matches your natural skin tone.

When testing different shades of foundation, bring your foundation down along the neck area, which tends to be lighter than the face. The jaw-line area will give you the best indication of whether or not the color is correct.

APPLY YOUR FOUNDATION—FLAWLESSLY

First things first: Make sure that before you apply your foundation, you use a make-up primer. I talked about primers in the Skincare section. They create a canvas for the foundation to go on smoothly. They will also extend the life of your foundation and keep it in place for hours. Find a primer you love and use it religiously!

People ask all the time about the best way to apply foundation. They don't know if they should be using their fingers, a sponge, or a brush. For liquid foundation, I highly recommend investing in a good foundation brush. I have never seen a professional make-up artist who knew what they were doing use anything else. A brush will allow the foundation to go on smoothly and evenly and will distribute just the right amount. A brush is also easy to wipe off and clean. A sponge holds dirt and bacteria, and so do your hands. You don't want those germs being transferred onto your face.

Celebrity make-up artist Jemma Kidd once gave me some great advice on the proper way to apply foundation. You don't smear foundation on like spackle!

Instead, you take your foundation brush and lightly press it into the skin. This will make sure you aren't applying too much color. She was right! I have applied my foundation this way ever since and I always get a flawless look.

Most importantly, when it comes to foundation, you want it to look like a second skin. You don't want to look like you are wearing anything at all. So make sure you are wearing a color that really blends in with your skin. When you find the right one, it will be almost invisible on your face.

But the right foundation in January won't necessarily be the right foundation in May! Just like we change our wardrobes from season to season, I also believe you need to make adjustments to your beauty wardrobe. I usually have two shades of foundation that I use—one for summer and one for winter. We tend to get a little darker in the summer just because we are exposed to the sun more often (I NEVER tan my face and always use an SPF, but your skin can still get a bit darker). The foundation I use in the summer is usually one to two shades darker than my winter foundation.

If you're like Stephanie and are looking for light coverage, tinted moisturizers also work well in the summertime when it is super hot and you feel like your make-up is going to slide right off your face. (I live in Texas and have witnessed this happening firsthand—NOT a pretty sight!) Just remember, they won't give you the same amount of coverage as a full foundation, so you might want to layer it with some translucent powder and, of course, concealer.

COUNT ON CONCEALER

Now that we've satisfied our foundation fix, the next step is concealer. Concealer is something EVERY woman should be using, especially around the nose, which can tend to be red, and under the eyes. It works best on areas that are discolored, like dark circles. A question commonly asked is, Which goes first? The foundation or the concealer? The answer is foundation first and concealer second. I can't stress enough the importance of a great concealer. Diamonds aren't the only things that are a girl's best friend! Find a concealer you love and have a life-long relationship with it. A concealer will always be there for you, especially in the bad times when you will count on it the most. I know my concealer has bailed me out countless times—late nights at work, little to no sleep, long nights out on the town, etc. The next morning is never pretty. A great concealer can breathe new life into your face, or at least help hide the damage you did the night before!

A good rule of thumb—choose a concealer that is two shades lighter than your natural skin tone. You don't want to go too light or it will look like you have white rings around your eyes, and if you go too dark, the concealer is not serving its purpose.

Just like you did with foundation, I also recommend you get color-matched for a good concealer. Ask the artist at the make-up counter for help in finding a good color for your skin. You really need to try it, especially with your foundation, to make sure that it works for you. And don't just take their word for it—grab a mirror and step into some natural light to make sure the color blends well with your skin.

I apply concealer with my ring finger, since it applies the least amount of pressure to that delicate skin area, and then I blend it with my foundation brush.

Concealer can really be used anywhere on your face. It's great for hiding blemishes. Just make sure that you don't pile on too much concealer over problem areas. That will cause more attention to the area you are trying to hide. The miracle concealer I talked about earlier is from Clé de Peau. This concealer has won every possible beauty award there is, and I can't live without it! It always disguises my dark circles, and people think I've slept for hours.

PERFECTLY PLACED POWDER

After I've applied my foundation and concealer, I usually like to follow it with a light dusting of translucent powder. Lancôme's Absolue powder is my favorite. This will help control shine and set your make-up. I like to use a loose powder and lightly dust it on my T-Zone area (forehead, nose, and chin). Don't use too much powder, or it will settle into fine lines and wrinkles. Just a light dusting is all you need.

If you still have a problem with shine control, try using a product like Lancôme's T-Zone Powder Gel for an instant fix. I often use this when I am on television, especially when I am under bright, hot lights. This product is amazing and really cuts down on shine. It is also oil-free. Apply it only in areas where you really need it—you won't need to use this product all over your face. I use it over my primer and before my foundation.

For touch-ups, I wouldn't recommend carrying a loose powder around with you. If it spills out, you're left with a huge mess. Instead, use a powder compact, or blotting papers work great, too. My favorite blotting papers are made by Shiseido.

HOW TO SPEND YOUR BEAUTY BUCKS—MY FAVORITE FOUNDATIONS AND CONCEALERS

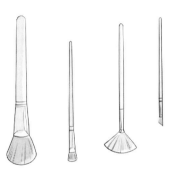

Full-Coverage Foundations

Elizabeth Arden Custom Color Foundation
Giorgio Armani Luminous Silk Foundation
Hourglass Veil Fluid Make-up
Lancôme Absolue Make-up
Laura Mercier Silk Crème Foundation
Laura Mercier Oil-Free Foundation
Le Métier de Beauté Peau Vierge

Sheer Foundation/Tinted Moisturizer

Chantecaille Just Skin Tinted Moisturizer
Giorgio Armani Face Fabric
Lancôme Teint Idole
Laura Mercier Tinted Moisturizer
YSL Teint Parfait Complexion Enhancer

Concealers

Clé de Peau Beaute Concealer
Dior Skinflash Radiance Booster Pen
Laura Mercier Secret Camouflage
YSL Touché Éclat

Translucent Loose Powders

Giorgio Armani Loose Powder
Lancôme Absolue Radiant Smoothing Powder
YSL Poudre Sur Mesure Semi-Loose Powder

Star Style

Victoria Beckham, a.k.a. Posh Spice, is probably one of the most fun celebrities to chat with. She is so open and really, really funny. I know you wouldn't think this because she rarely smiles in any of her pictures and always looks kind of miserable. But despite her perpetual pout, you have to admit—she always looks flawless! Her fashion taste is incredible and there's never a hair out of place on her head. I asked her to name her absolute favorite beauty product, one that she just couldn't live without. She told me it is Yves Saint Laurent's highlighter pen, Touche Eclat. Victoria says she uses it every day and loves it. Oh, and one more little fact about Victoria: She can also do a really fantastic, dead-on Donald Duck impression!

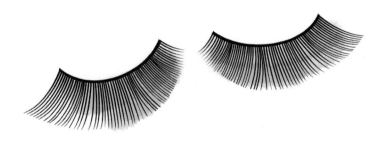

Question from Paula

My biggest make-up problem is that I keep getting eyeliner rubbing off onto my top lids. It doesn't usually happen right away but a few hours later, I look into the mirror and see an accidental Tammy Faye. Can you help me?

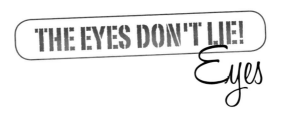

THE EYES DON'T LIE!
Eyes

The eyes are the windows to the soul. I'm not sure who first said that, but I really like it and I definitely believe it. When we engage in conversation, where do we look? The eyes, of course. If you really want to see what a person is feeling, look them dead in the eyes. The eyes don't lie. So, it makes sense that you want your eyes to be the focal point of your face. I like all eye shapes and colors. It's what makes your beauty distinct.

When it comes to beauty products, there are more items for your eyes than any other feature on your face—eye shadows, eyeliners, mascaras, highlighters. When I'm applying make-up, I always start with my eyes because I know this is the area where I will spend the most amount of time. I have big eyes, so I like to play them up. Sometimes I like a more natural look, or sometimes I feel like a dramatic smoky eye. It's fun to create and experiment with different looks.

Here are some of my very best tips for eyes. I will give them to you in the order that I apply my eye make-up.

EYE SHADOW BASICS

The very first product I put on my eyelid, even before I apply color, is an eye shadow primer. You've heard me use the P-word before. I don't like to repeat myself or waste anyone's time saying the same thing over and over and over. Obviously, this is important to me, and now it should be important to you. A good eye shadow primer will keep your shadow in place all day long.

Some people will use concealer or even foundation over their eyes to act as a primer. I find that creates a "thick" effect on my eyelids. A primer is nice and sheer and is specifically made to act as a smooth canvas for eye shadow application. It is worth the additional cost.

Just like for my foundation, I like to use a make-up brush to blend in my primer. You can also use your fingers, but I think a brush works better. I have a specific brush in my collection that is used *only* to apply my primer. It's important to be hygienic when you are working around your eyes, because bacteria can be transferred very easily. This could possibly lead to an eye infection, so you want to be careful.

After I've applied my primer, I apply my eyeliner. You may be thinking, wait a minute! Why isn't she applying her eye shadow next? There's a good reason. I learned a trick from a make-up artist a long time ago. She told me a thick line above your lashes is too harsh. Instead, she said to use a pencil eyeliner and draw my line above my lashes like normal. On the opposite side of your eyeliner, there is usually a blender. Take that and blend the eyeliner color about halfway up your eyelid. Then, apply your eye shadow. This will still give you the look of a darker line along your lashes, but it won't be a harsh line that stands alone. Of course, this trick will only work with dark eye shadows. If you are using a light eye shadow color, apply that first and then put your eyeliner on top. We'll discuss eyeliner in more detail below.

EYE SHADOW COLOR AND APPLICATION

The third time is the charm when it comes to eye shadow color, and I like to use three different colors. I start with a light shade that I apply all over my eye and bring up right underneath my brow bone. This creates the look of a highlighter, which helps open up the eyes. Then I apply a medium color all over my eyelid and finish up with a darker color in the contour area (the crease). You can use my eyeliner trick here too if you want. You would apply your light eye shadow color, and then your pencil eyeliner. After you smudge the color out, then you would apply your medium color over it. If you don't want to use the eyeliner trick, you would just apply your eyeliner after the contouring color. For the contour color, choose a shade that is in the same color family but a few shades darker.

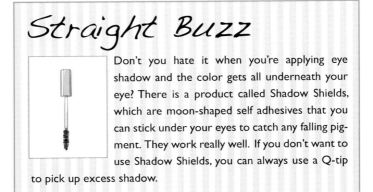

Straight Buzz

Don't you hate it when you're applying eye shadow and the color gets all underneath your eye? There is a product called Shadow Shields, which are moon-shaped self adhesives that you can stick under your eyes to catch any falling pigment. They work really well. If you don't want to use Shadow Shields, you can always use a Q-tip to pick up excess shadow.

I mentioned using a highlighter underneath the brow bone. I think this looks great and really opens up the eye area. I would even add a little on the inside corners of your eye to brighten that area as well.

Many women are unsure of what eye shadow palettes flatter them, so it's easy to play it safe and go with a basic brown color. But if you want to shake things up, go for an eye shadow shade that is the opposite of your eye color. If you have brown eyes, try a green, blue, or purple eye shadow color. If you have blue eyes, try a rich mocha brown color. If you have green eyes, purple would be a fun shade to try. Hazel eyes can try colors that look best on green-eyed and brown-eyed people. I would stick to lighter colors for day and darker ones at night. I have hazel eyes, so I usually wear a light brown color at work, but a deep rich purple at night. Bobbi Brown cosmetics has some gorgeous eye shadow colors that I love to use—one of my favorites is Black Plum.

Some people like to wear a cream-based eye shadow. I highly discourage using one if your eyelids get even the slightest bit oily. Talk about an oil slick right on your own face! The color will slide right off. If you are dead set on using a cream eye shadow, be sure and apply just a tiny bit of loose, translucent powder over it to help keep the color in place.

For a special occasion or around the holidays, I will sometimes layer a little shimmer shadow over my eye shadow color. This is fun to do for a little extra drama, but save it for special events—although who am I to discourage people from adding a little drama to their lives?

EYELINER

There are several different kinds of eyeliner: pencil, liquid, shadow-based, and gel. They all serve their purpose, and some look better than others (at least in my opinion). I prefer to use an eyeliner pencil. It goes on easily and precisely. Make sure the point on your pencil is sharp and then line the lid, working from the inside to the outside. Try to get as close to the lash line as possible.

If you line the top of your eyelid, you should also line the bottom. It gives a more finished, polished look.

If I don't have an eyeliner pencil handy, I will use a dark mocha or black eye shadow color as my eyeliner. This is easy to do. Just be sure and apply the shadow with an eyeliner brush. This type of brush is usually very thin, so it will be easy to get the color close to the lash line. You can even create a liquid effect by wetting the brush with water and then dipping it into the color.

Lots of ladies like that '60s cat-eye look of a liquid liner. I am not a huge fan of liquid liner, because it can be rather unforgiving. If you mess up or make a mistake, it's hard to correct. That's not to say it doesn't look good. Angelina Jolie almost always wears a liquid liner, and I think she always looks pretty darn amazing!

If you are going to wear a liquid liner, *don't* use it to line underneath your eye. That will look way too harsh. And only use it in the evenings. I think the look of a liquid liner is too much for daytime.

You may or may not have heard of a gel eyeliner. This is kind of a cross between an eyeliner pencil and a liquid liner. It goes on with the ease of a pencil but gives the effect of a liquid liner. Bobbi Brown makes an excellent gel eyeliner that I highly recommend trying.

When I'm creating a smoky, dramatic eye I like to use eyeliner everywhere! I will not only line the outside of my eye, but the inside as well. Because that area is so close to your actual eyeball, you want to make sure you are extra careful. To avoid Paula's problem, definitely use a waterproof eyeliner, since that area is moist and the color will come right off if you don't. Some artists will line the inner rim of your eye with a white pencil to create the illusion of a bigger eye. Rimmel cosmetics makes a great white eyeliner that you can pick up at the drugstore.

MASCARA

There are some things that I just won't leave the house without, and mascara is one of them (lip gloss and concealer are the others, FYI). In fact, I became so addicted to the look of mascara that I started getting eyelash extensions, so it always looks like I am wearing mascara (we'll talk about extensions in a bit).

There are so many different kinds of mascara on the market—ones that lengthen, volumize, thicken, separate, plump, and loads of other things. Look carefully at your lashes, decide what you need, and then choose a mascara that will help you get the look you want.

Mascaras come in different colors, but I'm old school and think black mascara looks best on everyone. I was never one for choosing a teal or purple mascara! Let's keep the '80s in the '80s, OK?!

Two important steps you must take before you even think about whipping out that wand: First, curl your lashes! This will make a HUGE difference. A good lash curler is your best beauty friend. It will make your eyes look huge and your lashes look long and luscious. Second, apply a mascara primer. Yes, that word again—primer. If you don't want raccoon eyes, apply a primer to your lashes. Your mascara will stay in place all day long.

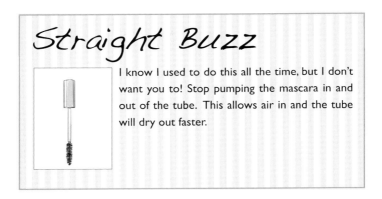

Straight Buzz

I know I used to do this all the time, but I don't want you to! Stop pumping the mascara in and out of the tube. This allows air in and the tube will dry out faster.

A couple of tricks for keeping your lashes curled—use your eyelash curler right after you get out of the shower or bath, when your lashes are still damp. They will hold their curl better. You can also try heating up your lash curler for just a few seconds with a warm hair dryer. Lightly blow some hot air on your curler, let it cool off briefly (you don't want to scald your lashes), and then curl your lashes with it. My favorite lash curler is by Shu Uemura, and it is the only one I will use (Madonna loves it, too). Others that I've tried hurt me, and I felt like I was going to rip my lashes out!

After you've prepped your lashes with your curler and primer, it's time to apply the mascara. Work from the base of your lashes to the tips. Wiggle the wand as you move it up your lash. Refrain from coating your lashes too many times, or you'll end up with clumps that are hard to separate.

I don't like to use any mascara at all on my bottom lashes. Mine are long, so it always reminded me of spider legs. I think it's overkill. If you use eyeliner on your bottom lash line, that should be plenty of color.

You can spend a lot of money on mascara, but I recommend against it. The reason—you should not keep a tube of mascara more than three or four months. Every time you open your tube, bacteria can get in, and that same bacteria can end up in your eye. That's why I recommend tossing the tube after a few months.

If you start tossing a pricey tube every three months, you're going to feel it in your Beauty Bucks wallet, but you can get a great mascara for less. I would say nine out of ten Hollywood make-up artists have a tube of Maybelline Great Lash in their kits. You know the one—it's that preppy pink and green mascara tube. They love it and use it on some of the biggest names in Tinseltown. It works *and* it's cheap. Buy it!

OTHER MASCARA OPTIONS— TINTING, FALSE LASHES, AND EXTENSIONS

Applying mascara can be a chore, and if you get tired of it you do have options. Lash tinting is one good way of getting that mascara look without actually applying any color at all. I would get it done in a reputable salon. It takes just a few minutes and the color lasts for three to four weeks.

If you're looking for length and volume, you have both home- and salon-based options: false lashes or lash extensions.

False lashes are all about glamour, and that's why women have been using them for decades. Shu Uemura makes the most amazing line of false lashes for women, and I like that they will teach you how to apply them yourself. Before you apply your lashes, make sure to curl your own. Whatever lashes you choose, hold them up to your eye. Chances are they are too long, so you will want to cut them to make sure they are the right size. Apply a very thin coat of glue to the lash band and apply them as close to your own lash line as possible. Finish the look with a coat of mascara. To remove them, simply start at the inner corner of your eye, and the lashes will peel right off. Any glue or residue left behind can easily be removed with cleanser or an oil-free remover.

If you really want a dramatic look, eyelash extensions are where it's at! You've heard of hair extensions, right? Just think of these as extensions for your lashes. A skilled lash artist will carefully apply the extensions to your lashes in a process that takes about an hour to an hour and a half. You don't have to curl them, and you don't wear any mascara. You need to get fills every two to three weeks. The extensions fall out with the natural shedding of your own lashes. I've had mine for over a year now and love having the look of mascara without spending a minute applying it!

HOW TO SPEND YOUR BEAUTY BUCKS—MY FAVORITE SHADOWS, EYELINERS, AND MASCARAS

Eye Shadows

Bobbi Brown eye shadow in Black Plum
Bobbi Brown eye shadow in Gunmetal
Bobbi Brown eye shadow in Hotstone
Bobbi Brown metallic cream shadow in Chrome Patina
Chanel Quadra eye shadow in Smoky Eyes
Chanel Quadra eye shadow in Spices
$ CoverGirl Eye Enhancers, in Café au Lait
Clé de Peau Eye Color Quad #11
Clé de Peau Eye Color Quad #20
Giorgio Armani eye shadow #15
Laura Mercier Eye Basics (primer)
$ L'Oréal Hip, Bright Shadow Duo in Reckless
MAC Blue My Mind
$ Maybelline Expert Wear eye shadow in Lasting Lilac
$ Maybelline Expert Wear eye shadow in Sunlit Bronze
Stila Kitten

Eyeliners

Bobbi Brown Long Wear Gel Eyeliner
Chanel Stylo Yeux Waterproof #10
Clé de Peau Intensifying Cream Eyeliner #103
$ CoverGirl Perfect Point Eye Pencil in Onyx
La Prairie Luxe Eye Definer
NARS Glitter Pencil B24
$ N.Y.C. New York Color Cosmetics Black Liner Pencil

Mascaras

$ CoverGirl Covergirl LashBlast in Very Black
Diorshow Mascara
Lancôme Cils Booster Super Enhancing Mascara
  Base (primer)
Lancôme Définicils
Lancôme Hypnôse Drama
$ Maybelline Falsies
$ Maybelline Great Lash Mascara in Very Black
$ Maybelline Lash Stiletto Ultimate Length Mascara in
  Very Black

Eyelash Curler

Shu Uemura Eyelash Curler (this is the only one I
  list because it is the only one you need!)

Star Style

I've interviewed countless Hollywood stars and I rarely get intimidated. But there was one actress who definitely made me feel a bit uneasy, and that was Angelina Jolie. I interviewed her during the height of her budding romance with Brad Pitt. The news of their relationship was just leaking and the press was going wild. I went to L.A. to interview her for their now infamous movie *Mr. and Mrs. Smith* and had no clue what she would be like with so much gossip and scandal surrounding her life. There were paparazzi swarming the hotel 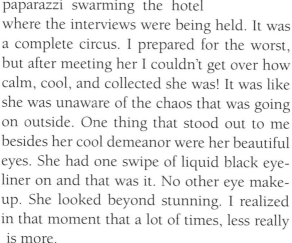 where the interviews were being held. It was a complete circus. I prepared for the worst, but after meeting her I couldn't get over how calm, cool, and collected she was! It was like she was unaware of the chaos that was going on outside. One thing that stood out to me besides her cool demeanor were her beautiful eyes. She had one swipe of liquid black eyeliner on and that was it. No other eye makeup. She looked beyond stunning. I realized in that moment that a lot of times, less really is more.

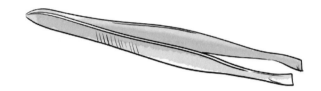

Question from Anne

I know you've talked about the importance of keeping your eyebrows groomed because they help frame your face. But I am having trouble finding a good product to make my eyebrows stand out because they are really light. Can you suggest a good product?

NO MORE CATERPILLARS
Eyebrows

When I think of eyebrows, two names pop into my head, and for very different reasons—Brooke Shields in the '80s (she's since discovered tweezers, thankfully) and Pamela Anderson. These are two women whose brows I have NEVER envied. I always thought Brooke Shields had the biggest, fuzziest eyebrows I'd ever seen, and they reminded me of caterpillars. Pamela Anderson, on the other hand, had brows that were so thin they looked like a straight line colored in with a brown pencil. You don't want either of these extremes. Something in the middle is just right.

If you don't believe me about the whole eyebrow thing, let me just let me say one name to you: Anastasia. If you don't know who I am talking about, this woman is a rock star in the world of eyebrows. She grooms every major star's eyebrows—from Madonna to Jennifer Lopez. Her salon in L.A. is the place to go for brow beauty. She's a wealthy woman because of her brow grooming technique and expertise. Do you believe me now?

It amazes me how many people simply ignore their brows. Maybe it's because they don't know how important they are. Your brows frame your face. This is a big deal. It's hard to hang up a picture without a picture frame, right? Stop neglecting your brows and let's pay some attention to them. Wait until you see the difference it makes!

BEAUTIFUL BROWS: GET SOME PROFESSIONAL HELP!

If you're a brow-grooming virgin, meaning you've never done anything to them before in the way of tweezing, waxing, cutting, brushing, etc., I want you to start doing some research. Think about all of your girlfriends. Who is the biggest groomer and the most concerned with her appearance? I'm sure you can guess who that is in my circle of friends! Find out where that friend goes to get her eyebrows groomed. More than likely, she is having them shaped professionally.

I think every woman at some point should seek out a professional and have her eyebrows shaped. I'm not saying you have to go back week after week, but at least get an idea of the shape they should be in. Once they are professionally shaped, it's easy to see where you need to tweeze as the new hair growth comes in.

Most eyebrow-waxing professionals will know exactly how to shape your brows once they see the shape of your face. That's why it's so important to get a good referral, because the good waxers know how to do this. If you don't have a referral, make sure to bring some pictures of the brows you want and don't be afraid to discuss the shape and style you are looking for. You certainly don't want to end up with pencil-thin brows when you wanted a more natural arch.

More than likely, your skin will turn slightly red after an eyebrow wax. This can last anywhere from thirty minutes to a couple of hours. I tend to schedule my brow waxing appointments for the end of the day when I know I can head straight home and not have to see anyone.

Of course, you could always try an at-home waxing kit. They sell these in most drugstores. I have never used one because, frankly, they make me nervous. I am very careful about what I put around my eye area. I would hate to get hot wax in my eye or, even worse, burn my skin. That's why I recommend leaving waxing to the professionals.

Threading is another way to groom your brows. It is an ancient method of hair removal that originated in Eastern countries like Egypt and India. A thin, twisted cotton thread is rolled over the hairs, removing them from the root. Since a larger area of hair is being re-moved at once, it can be quite painful. I have tried threading before and was not a fan! I found it to be too uncomfortable. But I also have girlfriends who love it. Try it for yourself and see which you prefer.

GROOMING YOUR BROWS AT HOME: UPKEEP

I always have the problem that my brows are super long. To keep them in shape, I take an eyebrow brush and brush all of my hairs upward. Whatever long, stray hairs I see, I make sure to cut them off at the top with a small pair of cuticle scissors so that they are the same length as my other brows.

There are a lot of eyebrow grooming kits that you can buy. They come with stencils and pencils and all kinds of other equipment. To be quite honest, I have no clue how to use those things. It's way too complicated for me! It's much easier to pick up the phone and make an appointment for a professional eyebrow shaping than it is to put a plastic stencil on my face, hold it steady, and attempt to shape my own brows. NO THANKS!

Follow a basic rule of thumb for eyebrow shaping: the beginning of your brow should be directly above the side of your nose. You can take a pencil or ruler or some other straight object and hold it from the side of your nose up to your eyebrow to make sure they are not starting too close in. To find out where your eyebrows end, use that same straight object and angle it from the outside corner of your eye. Any hairs that pass this point, tweeze.

Speaking of tweezing, you *must* have a good pair of tweezers. This is essential unless you like the look of a unibrow! I think Tweezerman makes the best pair of tweezers. You want something with a rounded tip, and nothing too pointy, which can be dangerous. I've stabbed myself plenty of times with a sharp-pointed pair of tweezers, and trust me, you don't want that to happen to you.

OTHER BROW BEAUTY FIXES

To answer Anne's question, a brow pencil is probably the easiest way to add some color to your brows. Just make sure that you aren't drawing a harsh line, or it will look like you are drawing on your brows rather than subtly bringing them out. This is that "Pam Anderson" look I was talking about.

Straight Buzz

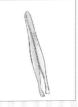

Make sure that when you are tweezing, you pull the hair in the direction of its growth. If you go against the growth, you will get ingrown hairs. Ouch! If you don't own a magnifying mirror, it's easiest to spot the hairs in natural light, so move whatever mirror you do have over to a window and get to work.

You can also use some eye shadow along with a brow brush to give your brows some color and definition. I find this difficult to do, so I just stick with a pencil.

I always finish up with a brow gel. I have lots of unruly eyebrows that love to go in all sorts of different directions. A brow gel is the only thing that will keep them in place. Just use a light touch when applying it, or the gel can get thick and harden.

If you're changing your hair color, don't forget to ask your stylist to dye your brows to match. Isn't it just so weird when you see a blonde with dark brown eyebrows? My sister is a brunette with naturally blonde eyebrows, so she is always dyeing them to match or using a darker brow pencil.

Finally, there is always that chance of a brow disaster happening. That's why it's important to get a good waxing or threading referral, talk with the professional prior to the appointment, and watch what they are doing with a hand-held mirror. If you feel like the wax is too hot or too much hair is being plucked out, SAY SOMETHING! Always be specific about what you want.

If something bad does happen, head straight to your nearest department store and seek out a make-up artist you trust. That artist can show you how to properly apply a brow powder or pencil to hide the mistake until your own brows can grow back in.

HOW TO SPEND YOUR BEAUTY BUCKS—MY FAVORITE EYEBROW PRODUCTS

Eyebrow Gels

Anastasia Brow Gel
Dior Brow Gel
MAC Brow Finisher
Victoria's Secret PRO Brow FX Grooming Gel

Eyebrow Pencils

Anastasia Perfect Brow Pencil
Dior Diorshow Brow Styler Ultra-Fine Precision
 Brow Pencil
LORAC Creamy Brow Pencil
$ Maybelline Define-A-Brow Eyebrow Pencil

Eyebrow Powders

Anastasia Brow Powder Duo
Benefit Smokin' Eyes/Sexy Eye and Brow Makeover
 Kit
LORAC Take A Brow

Tweezers

$ Revlon Slant Tip Expert Tweezer
Tweezerman Slant Tweezer

Star Style

Rene Russo is a stunning actress who seems to be defying the laws of aging. She is one of the rare people in this world who truly seems to get better with age. When I had the privilege of interviewing her, I just had to ask what her beauty secret was. She told me about a product that I had never heard of before: Frownies. She told me Frownies are like Botox in a box. They are little strips of paper that you moisten and put on your face wherever you have lines and wrinkles. The company claims that the product can help reduce wrinkles while you sleep. I don't know if it's the Frownies or just good genes, but whatever Rene is doing, keep it up, girl! You look amazing!

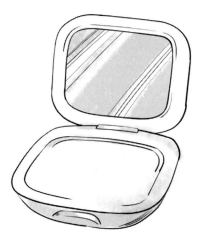

Question from Shelby

I'm not sure that I am applying my blush correctly. It ends up looking more like two red circles on my cheeks. Do you have any tips for making my blush look more natural?

CLOWN FACE BE GONE!
Cheeks

Can anyone say clown face? Come on, admit it! I know I'm not alone. You've been guilty of this before. You put way too much blush on your cheeks and the next thing you know, all you can see are those big red round circles. I so can relate to this. All I have to do is look at my old high school prom picture, and I am sorely reminded of just how clueless I was about make-up application. Besides the white feather dress I wore (no joke), the only other thing you can see in that picture are my clown cheeks. Good Lord! What was I thinking!?

Blush is supposed to make you look like you have a natural flush. You know, the way you look when you've come in from the cold or maybe just finished a run. Blush is supposed to give you a healthy, young, vibrant glow. You want to add some color, but nothing that looks unnatural.

GET CHEEKY!

Choosing the right shade is the most important step to getting that healthful glow. If you have pale skin like me, use a light pink color like Bobbi Brown's Pink Sugar. For medium skin tones, coral or peach looks great, and darker skin tones can get away with a rich rose color. Remember, the key with blush is to make it look as natural as possible, so when in doubt, just remember that less is always more.

I like to use a powder blush because I think it is the easiest to apply. To make sure you are applying it in the right place, look into a mirror, smile, and notice where the apples of your cheeks are. That's where you want to apply your blush.

Use a blush brush to apply the color to your cheeks. Always remember to tap off any excess powder. This will ensure you aren't putting on too much color. Then use a light sweeping motion to apply the color to the apples of your cheeks.

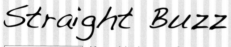

Straight Buzz

Keep blush away from your eye area and resist the urge to use it on your nose, forehead, or around the hairline. It will make you look uneven and too heavily made-up.

You don't want to stop the color just there. Blend some of it up at an angle but make sure the majority of the color is staying on your cheeks. The key word here is BLEND. If you don't, you'll look like you have two stripes on your face. Also, don't put loose powder on over your blush. Your powder should go on before your blush. If you've applied too much blush, use a tissue to gently wipe off the excess.

Another way to make sure you don't end up with clown face: apply your blush using natural light. In fact, this is a great way to apply any make-up. If you don't have a make-up mirror with the daytime light setting, make sure to sit by a window and use natural light when applying your make-up. There's no way you will apply too much color this way.

There are several blush options for those who don't like a powder blush. Some women prefer to use a cream blush. This works well for people with dry or normal skin, but not for those with oily skin. The color will slip right off. Cream blush is best applied with your fingers, since it really needs to be blended into the skin. I find this is easier to do with my fingers than with a brush.

Have you ever tried to use a cheek stain? That's another option, but I'm not crazy about those. I don't know about you but I just can't seem to apply it correctly. It ends up drying so fast on my face that I never have time to properly blend it. I end up with a weird-looking dot on my cheek. If you like cheek stains and know how to apply them, more power to you! I'll pass.

Finally, NARS cosmetics makes a great product called The Multiple. It's a multi-purpose cream-based stick for cheeks, lips, and eyes. I like to use a little dab of it on the apples of my cheeks. It gives a nice healthy glow. This is more of a highlighter, so you'll want to use it over your powder blush to add a hint of color, instead of using it alone. It is cream-based, so it will work best on ladies with normal and dry skin.

HOW TO SPEND YOUR BEAUTY BUCKS—MY FAVORITE CHEEK COLORS

Blush

Armani Beauty Sheer Blush
Bobbi Brown Pink Sugar
Chantecaille Aquablush
Lancôme Oil-Free Powder Blush
NARS Blush in Orgasm and Super Orgasm
NARS The Multiple in Orgasm
Shu Uemura Glow On Blush

Star Style

This probably won't come as a surprise to anyone, but Halle Berry is insanely gorgeous. I mean, the woman does not have a visible pore on her face! If you think she looks stunning in magazines and pictures, she is even more unbelievably beautiful in person. When I interviewed her I just had to know what kind of make-up she was using. I was expecting her to say some kind of expensive beauty line. It's not like she can't afford it! But no, she told me she stands behind Revlon. Halle has been a spokesperson for Revlon for years. She told me she supports the company because she really loves their products and believes in them. How refreshing is that!?

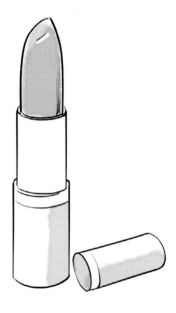

Question from Corinne

I always seem to have a problem with keeping my lipstick in place. Do you know of any product or primer that can help keep my lipstick where it belongs?

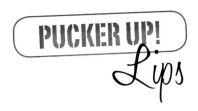

PUCKER UP!
Lips

OK, so I have to admit it. I've been waiting until now to tell you. When it comes to lipstick and lip gloss, I have a bit of a problem. I have a bit of an addiction to all things gloss. It's probably more of an obsession. I LOVE LOVE LOVE lip gloss. I don't know what it is, but I can never have enough of it. I probably have about fifteen tubes with me in my handbag at all times. Is this weird? Please tell me you do, too?! OK, you don't have to. It's all right. But I really do love lip gloss. Whenever I'm having a bad day, for some reason, a new lip gloss just makes me feel better. And it's a heck of a lot cheaper than a new pair of shoes if I need a retail pick-me-up!

When it comes to lipstick, the most common question I get is, How do I keep my lipstick on? It really is a big problem. I know I hate that gross lipstick mark I leave on a glass after drinking. There is only one person I know who can really keep her lipstick on through a meal, through drinking, through just about everything. That's my sister, Jennifer. I don't know how she does it. My mom and I laugh about it all the time. But I have seen the girl take as long as five minutes painstakingly applying her lip liner, lipstick, and then gloss. Maybe that's the key—you have to put in some time!

GET YOUR GLOSS ON

You know I love to tell it to you like it is—so don't leave the house without your lip gloss or lipstick or whatever you like best.

I don't follow the same lip color routine every day. Some days I feel like just wearing some lip gloss. Other days I put on lipstick and gloss. And then there are days I wear lip liner, lipstick, and lip gloss. It all depends on my mood and the occasion, but you can bet I am wearing something. You don't always have to use three products on your lips at all times (unless you are going somewhere fancy and important), so just go with the flow of the day. If you're not going to put on any make-up at all, at least apply a bit of balm so it looks like you tried!

LIPSTICK DO'S AND DON'TS: TIPS AND TRICKS FOR A PRETTY POUT

Before I start with any of my best lipstick tips, we HAVE to talk about a MAJOR pet peeve of mine. It's the dark liner/light lipstick faux pas. I can't stand this look! If you're doing this, PLEASE STOP! It's not a good look and is completely unnatural. Your lip liner should never be several shades darker than your lipstick. You want those two products to complement each other and contribute to an overall polished look, not become a distracting focal point. Choose a lip liner that is in the same color family as your lipstick. You want it to be just a few shades darker than your lipstick or gloss.

Since we're on the topic of pet peeves, I do have one more. I promise this is the last one! DON'T match your lipstick color to your outfit. This look is so dated. You want to wear a lipstick color that best flatters your skin tone and not your blouse!

Of course, it's not all about the color! You also want your lips to be pucker perfect, but chapped lips, lines around the mouth, and thin lips create common lip color obstacles for many woman. Luckily, I have easy fixes for all three!

Straight Buzz

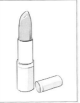

One of the most embarrassing things ever is walking around with lipstick on your teeth. Ugh! And I especially hate when no one tells you! HELP A GIRL OUT and speak up if you see someone with lipstick on her teeth! To make sure you never have to deal with the embarrassment, here is a trick. After you apply your lipstick and/or gloss, take your index finger, put it in your mouth, hold your lips around it, and then pull it out. All of that excess color will end up on your finger instead of your teeth. Yay!

First, your lip products will never go on smoothly if you have dry, chapped lips. You have to exfoliate your lips just like you exfoliate your skin. There are plenty of products out there that you can spend money on to help you exfoliate. But I say, forget those! Just take a washcloth one or two times a week and lightly rub your lips. It will help remove any dry, dead skin.

I always apply a lip balm before I go to sleep every night. I keep it in my nightstand. I have used Jo Malone's Vitamin E Lip Conditioner for years. It is incredibly hydrating and nourishing, and will help fight chapped lips before they start.

Lots of ladies also write to me complaining about lines around their lips. Those lines create that "bleeding" and feathering look. Try using a lip primer treatment before you put on your lipstick. It will not only help with lipstick feathering and bleeding, it keeps the lipstick in place for a longer period of time. MAC cosmetics makes one called MAC Prep and Prime Lip Treatment that I use daily. Since lip gloss can make its way into these lines even more easily than lipstick, you might want to consider using a shimmer lipstick. It will still give you the shine of a gloss without having to use one.

Finally, plumped-up lips are still a look a lot of women like to achieve. I've tried plenty of "lip plumping" lipsticks before, and I have to tell you, I'm not impressed. Sure, they work (and sting like crazy) for about two or three minutes after you apply them, but after that, I couldn't tell a difference. I'm not a fan. If you really want that bee-stung look, talk to a doctor about lip fillers like Restylane and Juvéderm.

However, there is a trick you can do to make your lips look bigger than they really are without paying a doctor for injections. Make-up artists have done this on me before and I think it works well. Take a nude lip liner and line just outside your natural lip line. Fill in the color all over your lips, and then finish with lipstick and gloss. Your lips will instantly look fuller.

CHOOSING A SHADE

I personally love a nude lip color. Nudes are universally flattering and much easier to apply than a dark, deep red lipstick. In fact, dark lipsticks can age a woman—if you look at a picture of a woman with dark lip color and then the same woman in a nude or light pink lip color, it is astounding how much better a lighter lip color looks. It takes YEARS off!

If you do love that red lipstick, there is certainly nothing wrong with it. It's Gwen Stefani's go-to-color and her signature trademark. She looks gorgeous in it. If you do wear red lip color, go light on the eyes. I wouldn't do heavy eye make-up. You will look too heavily made up. But remember that choosing the right shade of red depends on your skin tone! If you have a warm skin tone, orange-reds look best, while people with cool undertones should choose a blue-red shade. Of course, you can never go wrong with a rich, classic red.

Just like liquid liner, red lipstick is unforgiving in its application. If you mess up, believe me, you can tell! Definitely use a liner first, apply the lipstick, and then dust your lips lightly with some translucent powder to set the color. Top it off with gloss and you should be good to go!

If your lipstick does smudge, grab a Q-tip to clean up the area. If there is still some excess color on the skin around your mouth, put a dab of concealer over it to cover the pigment and even out your skin tone.

My listeners also ask if they should line before or after applying their lipstick. I've seen make-up artists do it both ways. I don't think there is one right way and one wrong way. It's a personal preference. I personally like to lightly line my lips before my lipstick. Then, I use my index finger to blend in the color from the lip liner all over my lips, making sure the color covers the entire lip area. Finish the look with lipstick and gloss.

Straight Buzz

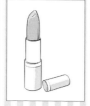

Just like your skin, lips can also be exposed to potential sun damage. You want to make sure they are protected, so if you can find products that contain an SPF, use them!

Whatever color you go with, you won't want to be reapplying it all day—but have you ever actually tried those long-lasting or long-wearing lipsticks that promise to stay in place for at least eight hours? I HATE those things! They totally dry my lips out. I've tried several different brands and they all feel awful on the lips. I don't use them and I don't think you will like them either!

If you take the time to properly apply your lipstick with a lip liner, you can make it last without having to buy these long-wear lipsticks. Just how long your lipstick lasts depends on you. If you drink a lot of water, coffee, soft drinks, etc. throughout the day, your lipstick is not going to last as long. I certainly want you to stay hydrated, so I'm not telling you to stop drinking fluids. The best advice is to use a lip liner, which tends to stay on longer than a lipstick or gloss. Or trying using a straw when you drink—less product will come off your lips when you drink through a straw.

So, to wrap it up: If you're like Corinne and want to keep your lipstick lasting longer, the best way is to use a lip liner and apply it as I've explained above. That way, if your lipstick does wear off, you have some color left from your liner.

HOW TO SPEND YOUR BEAUTY BUCKS—MY FAVORITE LIP PRODUCTS

Lip Balms and Primers

Jack Black Intense Therapy Lip Balm
Jo Malone Vitamin E Lip Conditioner
MAC Prep and Prime Lip Treatment
$ Olay Regenerist Lip Anti-Aging Concentrate
Rhonda Allison Eye and Lip Repair Serum
$ Rosebud Salve

Lip Liners

Bobbi Brown Slopes
Chanel Nude
Chantecaille Tone
Lancôme Sheer Raspberry
Laura Mercier Clover
MAC Spice
MAC Subculture
NARS Papua

Lipsticks

Giorgio Armani Silk #14
Lancôme Color Fever Shine New Year's Resolution
MAC Cremesheen Crème D'Nude
NARS Belle de Jour
NARS Honolulu Honey
NARS Viva Las Vegas

$ Neutrogena Moisture Shine Lipstick SPF 20
Tom Ford Blush Nude
Tom Ford Ginger Fawn
Tom Ford True Coral
YSL Rouge Volupté

Lip Glosses

By Terry Laque de Rose—Rose Kiss
By Terry Laque de Rose—Sinful Rose
By Terry Rose Balm
Chanel Glossimer #121
Chanel Glossimer #139
Chanel Glossimer #146
Giorgio Armani Lip Shimmer #1
Giorgio Armani Lip Shimmer #25
Laura Mercier Rose
MAC Lipglass C-Thru
MAC Lipglass Prrr
MAC Plushglass Big Baby
NARS Greek Holiday
NARS Turkish Delight
YSL Golden Gloss
YSL Gloss Pur

Star Style

It's hard not feeling like a giant Amazon next to Nicole Richie. She is so tiny, but her personality is huge and full of life. I got a chance to talk to her about her clothing line, Winter Kate. She is a great designer. When I interviewed her, I noticed that she didn't have a lot of make-up on. She told me she really hates to wear a lot of make-up and is more likely not to be wearing any at all. (I'm sure that has a lot to do with the fact that she is now a mom to two adorable kids!) In fact, when I asked her what her favorite must-have beauty product was, she told me she didn't have one at all. I couldn't believe it! Doesn't everyone have at least one product they just can't live without? She insisted that she didn't. But then I looked over her shoulder and noticed a lip gloss sticking out her handbag. It was a Chanel Glossimer. I couldn't make out the color, but I asked her if that might be a product she really liked. I finally got her to say yes!

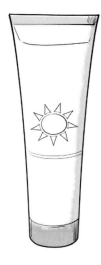

Question from Maggie

I am starting to think about getting a tan for summer. I really don't want to tan in a tanning bed anymore. Are there any good self-tanners or lotions that actually work without leaving streaks, won't turn me orange, and won't make me stink of some strange smell?

UNLEASH YOUR INNER GOLDEN GODDESS!
Bronzers

It's one thing to have that beautiful porcelain skin in the winter, but when summer rolls around, I want to look like a golden goddess. There is no way I am basking in the sun to get that glow, and you better not be either! We are way too smart for that. No one wants cancer, for crying out loud! There are so many SAFE ways to get a great-looking tan. If you have a membership to some tanning bed place, CANCEL IT! Those things are scary and look like coffins with heated-up lightbulbs. Gross! Let's get a safe tan we can all feel good about.

BRONZED BEAUTY: FAUX-TANNING YOUR BODY

The key to a great, natural-looking tan is exfoliation! You MUST exfoliate before you even think about applying a self-tanning cream or getting a spray tan.

Be sure to exfoliate your face *and* your body, paying particular attention to places that tend to be more dry—elbows, knees, tops of your heels. And definitely shave your legs and underarms BEFORE applying a self-tanning cream. You don't want to shave these areas after your self-tanner is applied, or you will run the risk of some of the color coming off with the razor.

Lots of people recommend that you wear gloves when you apply your self-tanning lotion. I never do and I don't have a problem with streaking. Just make sure you know where you're applying the color and wash your hands thoroughly after application so you don't get those telltale orange palms.

I like to apply my self-tanning cream in long, even strokes, starting with my legs and working my way up the body. On my legs, I smooth the cream downward, making sure I cover all areas. I continue the strokes downward on my arms and across my chest and stomach. You should always read the specific instructions on the bottle, but make sure to give yourself ten to fifteen minutes before getting dressed. It's important to let the tanner dry so it won't stain your clothes.

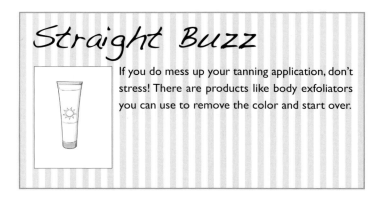

Straight Buzz

If you do mess up your tanning application, don't stress! There are products like body exfoliators you can use to remove the color and start over.

If you're still worried about applying the correct amount in an even way, try using tanning towelettes. They are kind of like "Tanning for Dummies." You only need one towelette for your entire body, and the color always comes out evenly for me. I like that you don't have to guess how much product to use. It's all right there on one towelette. My favorite tanning towelette is by skincare expert Kate Somerville.

Of course, you can also make an appointment at a salon and get a professional to give you that sun-kissed radiance. But you know I am going to be FURIOUS if you are still using a tanning bed. Get out of it! Try a spray tan or an airbrush tan instead. It is much safer and you will still get an amazing color.

There is a difference between a spray tan and an airbrush tan. A spray tan is something you would get inside a booth with a machine. The machine blasts you with color as you rotate your body in different directions. An airbrush tan is applied by a person who uses a kind of "gun" to spray color on you. This is much more precise because it is being applied by an actual person, and I think the overall effect is far superior to a spray tan. Because of this, an airbrush tan usually costs more than a regular spray tan. Since it is pricey, you might want to save the airbrush tanning appointment for special occasions like a wedding, class reunion, important dinner date, etc.

You should wait to shower or bathe at least six to eight hours after receiving an airbrush or spray tan treatment. It takes that long for the color to fully develop. Don't go and work out after a sunless tan, or you'll watch the color run right off your skin along with your sweat!

Most airbrush and spray tan treatments come in shades to match your skin tone—usually light, medium and dark. If you have fair skin, don't choose dark. It will be way too much color and could look very fake.

I have fair skin and usually choose the light or medium options. You want to add a few shades of color that makes it look like you've been spending some time in the sun. You don't want to look like a pale white ghost one day, and then the next, like you've spent a week in the desert without any sunscreen.

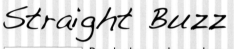

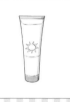

People always ask me what to apply first, powder bronzer or blush. You should apply your bronzer first and then a light application of blush right on the apples of your cheeks.

Most salons also offer a tanning service where they will exfoliate your body from head to toe and then apply a self-tanning lotion. This is a great service if you can afford it.

The biggest complaint about self-tanning products is their smell. It's hard to describe exactly what that scent is, but I do know it's strange and funky, just like Maggie said! When you go out self-tanner shopping, choose products from the list I've provided at the end of this section. I've tried them all and none of them stink. If there's one you want to try that's not on the list, open the cap and smell it first.

GET THAT GLOW: APPLYING BRONZER TO YOUR FACE

To get a great glow on my face, I sometimes like to mix liquid bronzers with my moisturizer or foundation. Use slightly less than the normal amount of product you normally would and then add just a tiny drop of a liquid bronzer. Apply the foundation with your make-up brush as usual. This will give your face a nice, natural, sun-kissed glow. Just be sure not to go overboard with your product. Less really is more here, and you certainly don't want to look like a giant pumpkin head!

I also like using powder bronzers on my face. I think any skin tone can use them—from fair to dark. I use them year-round. I just make sure to use less in the winter than I do in the summer so it doesn't look unnatural. My favorite powder bronzers are by NARS and Bobbi Brown because I think they look the most natural.

When you apply your bronzer, you want to hit three main areas—along the sides of your forehead, along the cheekbone, and just under the jaw-line. Do not apply powder bronzer on your nose, in the middle of your forehead, or on your chin.

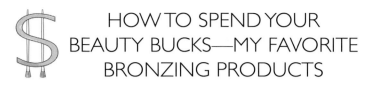

HOW TO SPEND YOUR BEAUTY BUCKS—MY FAVORITE BRONZING PRODUCTS

Body Exfoliators

Bliss Fatgirl Scrub
Kate Somerville's ExfoliKate Body
Sisley Energizing Foaming Exfoliant for the Body

Body Bronzers

Estée Lauder Sunless Super Tan
Kate Somerville 360 Tanning Towelettes
Lancôme Flash Bronzer
$ L'Oréal Sublime Bronze
MAC To the Beach Bronze Body Oil
NARS Body Glow
$ Nivea Sun-Kissed Firming Moisturizer
Scott Barnes Body Bling
St. Tropez Bronzing Mousse

Powder Bronzers (Face):

Estée Lauder Bronze Goddess Soft Duo Bronzer
Giorgio Armani Sheer Bronzer
Lancôme Star Bronzer
NARS Bronzing Powder

Liquid Bronzers (Face):

Fresh High Noon Freshface Glow
MAC Lustre Drops

YSL Teint Parfait Complexion Enhancer "Colour Booster" shades

Star Style

Kate Somerville is *the* facialist to the stars. When Hollywood celebrities need to look red-carpet ready, they head straight to her skincare clinic in L.A. Fortunately, for those of us who can't fly to California to see her, Kate does have a fantastic line of skincare products. But her top seller isn't a serum or moisturizer. It's her tanning towelettes. When I had the opportunity to meet her, she told me that those tanning towelettes were specifically formulated for one of her best clients—Paris Hilton. Kate was so tired of Paris coming into her clinic with bad orange faux tans that she developed a product just for the socialite that would give her a much more natural glow. I never thought I would say it, but "Thanks, Paris!"

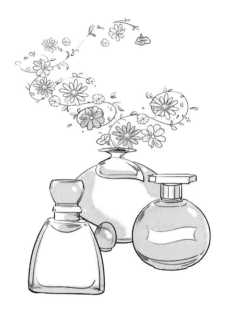

Question from Katie

I love wearing perfume, but I always feel like the minute I put it on the smell is gone. Is there a way to make my fragrance last longer?

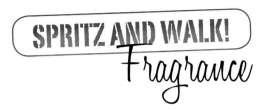

SPRITZ AND WALK!
Fragrance

Who hasn't stepped onto an elevator early in the morning half-asleep, only to be quickly woken up by the startling smell of way-too-strong perfume? You know what I mean. It's the scent that just lingers and seems to make its home right up your nose. A headache starts to form in your temples, and the smell is something that just won't go away. For the woman who is bathing in her fragrance, PLEASE STOP! There is no reason to use half the bottle in one single day. Your fragrance is meant to last more than a week, so seriously, calm down with the spritzing.

Fragrance is supposed to be a good thing, an alluring scent that is so personal that when people smell it, they instantly think of you. I have worn what I call my signature scent for years—Jo Malone's Red Roses. I adore the fragrance and wear it daily. Sometimes I will switch it up for fun, but nine times out of ten, I am wearing my Red Roses.

I have always found that one of the most frustrating things is when you notice an amazing perfume on someone else—and when you try it on your own skin, it smells totally different! It's so disappointing, because we want it to smell just as good on us. But because of our bodies' different oils and chemical make-up, not all fragrances are created equal. The bottom line is, you have to find something that smells amazing on you!

PROPER PERFUME APPLICATION

There is an easy way to ensure that you are never the woman in the elevator who is stinking the place up! I call it the "Spritz and Walk." To get the perfect amount of perfume, spritz two pumps of scent in the air and walk through the cloud of fragrance. You'll be covered head to toe in fragrance, but nothing too overwhelming. That way, people will get a captivating whiff as you walk by, not start sneezing!

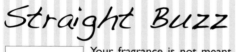

Straight Buzz

Your fragrance is not meant to last forever, so make sure to use it before you lose it. Most perfumes will only last a year or two tops. To get the most out of it, store it in a cool, dark area and away from direct sunlight. Keep the cap on tightly.

I also don't think there is anything wrong with spraying a little fragrance in your hair. It might sound strange, but I always tend to get compliments when I spritz just a small amount on the back of my head.

If you still think it is absolutely necessary to spray perfume on your wrists, go for it. Just make sure not to rub them together after you spray your fragrance there. That will change the scent and diminish its full effect.

The question I get asked the most about perfume is how to make the scent last (which is probably why so many women over-spritz in the morning: to avoid the afternoon fade). When I really love a fragrance, it is all about layering for me. I like to use a body lotion with that same scent or even a body oil or scented soap.

I also like the trick of using Vaseline to keep your fragrance lasting longer. Just dab a bit of Vaseline on your arm or on the back of your neck and spritz a little fragrance right on top. The Vaseline will help keep the scent lingering longer—fixing Katie's problem and making her perfume last throughout a workday or a night on the town!

However, don't spray your perfume in areas like under your arms, in your chest area, or behind your ears. Your natural body scent in these areas won't mix well with your perfume.

Finally, if you really want to get your perfume's full effect, don't wear a lot of competing scents: things like scented deodorants or body creams and body oils that are not from the same line as your fragrance. These scents are basically doing battle with each other, but in this fight, no one wins.

PICKING YOUR SIGNATURE SCENT

It's all about trial and error when you're trying to find that perfect perfume. Head to your favorite department store and test out what they have to offer. Fragrances are usually separated into different categories like floral, fruity, citrus, musk, woodsy, and sporty scents. You should have an idea of what scents you personally like. You can also ask the salesperson behind the counter for a sample to take home—that way you can test it out for a few days and see if it's a scent that works for you.

Age can also play a factor in fragrance choice. Most young girls choose sweeter scents like vanilla. As they mature, women usually like to wear a more sophisticated scent like the legendary Chanel No. 5.

The time of year can also play a role in our perfume preference. Seasonal scents for fall and winter are usually heavy, spicy, and aromatic and commonly include amber and musk. During spring and summer, we enjoy fresh-smelling fragrances like delicate florals and fruits.

There are so many different types and prices that it can be hard to tell the difference between qualities of perfume. Here is a basic breakdown:

- Parfum—the most expensive and the scent will last the longest (you do get what you pay for here)
- Eau de Parfum—this has less oil and won't last as long as a Parfum
- Eau de Toilette—subtle fragrance
- Eau de Cologne—this is the least expensive and has the weakest scent

When you test a perfume, don't smell it right away. Wait a few seconds and wave the test paper in the air for a bit. If you smell it right away, you will get a big whiff of alcohol and not much else. This is because you are only smelling the perfume's top note. A perfume has three sets of notes. The top note is the first scent you smell after applying the perfume. The middle note is the main body of the perfume. Finally, the base note brings depth to the fragrance and usually is not noticed until at least thirty minutes after application.

Wear the fragrance around for a while. If you are out shopping, head to the fragrance counter first and put some product on. Walk around for a while and see if you get any reactions from people (other than from the counter person who is telling you how AMAZING you smell). I am sure you do, but it's always nice to get some unsolicited compliments.

HOW TO SPEND YOUR BEAUTY BUCKS—MY FAVORITE FRAGRANCE LINES

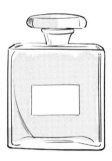 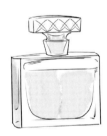

Child—cult favorite among major Hollywood celebs created by Dallas-based perfumer Susan D. Owens

Creed—amazing fragrances for both women and men

Fresh—if you have a sweet tooth, Brown Sugar is delicious!

Issey Miyake

Jo Malone—this British line is great for women and men

L'Artisan Parfumeur

Quelques Fleurs

Tom Ford Beauty

Star Style

Kate Beckinsale is so gorgeous and one of my favorite Hollywood actresses. I interviewed her for the film *Underworld*, and the minute I stepped inside the interview suite, I instantly smelled the most amazing scent. I had to ask her what it was. She told me it was actually a body oil called Sage Onyx perfume oil that she had worn for years. It smelled incredible! Of course, the minute I was finished with the interview, I rushed out to find this intoxicating fragrance. To my dismay, it didn't smell nearly as good on me as it did on her (not surprising). But it taught me that it is totally worth it to continue that search for your perfect scent.

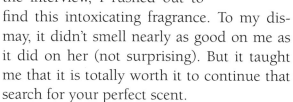

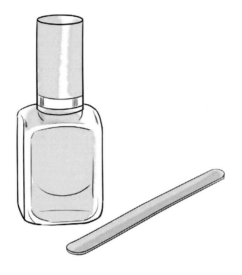

Question from Carrie

I was wondering what you like better—a cuticle cream or cuticle oil?

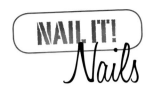

NAIL IT!
Nails

I don't know what it is about us ladies, but we sure do love our manis and pedis. Keeping our nails looking great makes sense. We do everything with our hands—we talk with them, type with them, write with them, make meals with them, make calls with them, wash dishes with them, shake hands with them. The list is endless.

I'm not sure about you, but I always pay attention to a person's nails. I have seen so many beautiful, well-kempt women who are perfectly dressed with flawless hair and make-up, and then I look down and what do I see—chipped nails. Keeping your nails in good shape can take time, but it doesn't have to be costly. Many of us can't afford a weekly manicure and pedicure, and that is perfectly fine. I have some tips on ways to keep your nails looking great and like you just stepped out of the salon.

HOW TO GET HEALTHY NAILS

It's a fact that what you eat can make a big difference in the health of your nails. Daily doses of foods that contain vitamins, minerals, and enzymes will help you maintain strong, healthy nails. Foods rich in zinc and vitamin B, like fresh carrot juice and broccoli, will help strengthen your nails. Dairy products rich in calcium are also good for nail strengthening. A lack of vitamin A, B_{12}, and calcium can cause dryness and brittleness, while a lack of protein, folic acid, and vitamin C can cause hangnails. Sometimes it's hard to work in all the nutrients you should, but at the very least, pop a multivitamin once daily!

There are a lot of products on the market designed to strengthen nails. I do believe these work to a point. They certainly can't hurt, but I'm not convinced they are worth the money. I have always found that when I am eating a healthy, clean diet of fruits, vegetables, and proteins, my nails grow like weeds and are super strong.

Even great nutrition doesn't guarantee picture-perfect hands, though; external factors can also keep your hands from looking their best. The harsh chemicals involved in normal household chores like doing dishes, laundry, and house cleaning can wreak havoc on your nails, so protect your hands with gloves whenever you can.

I like to keep my nails relatively short and neat. I think this style is easy to maintain and looks the most natural. It is a personal preference, but I don't think super-long nails look very professional. I would keep them no longer than half an inch past your fingertips.

NAIL POLISH TIPS

Cutting your own nails can be tricky, so I prefer to file them down with an emery board. The nail is much easier to shape this way. I prefer a square nail with the corners rounded in more of an oval shape. I used to have my nails filed straight across the top and sides, but often found that they broke much easier and faster that way.

When I get a professional manicure, the manicurist often tries to cut my cuticles. This can lead to hangnails. Don't try and cut your own cuticles. Instead, use a cuticle softener and then push them back with a cuticle pusher.

If you are doing your own nails, always start with a base coat. This will help strengthen and protect the nail bed. Next, apply two coats of your favorite nail polish color. Wait a few minutes and then finish with a top coat. A top coat will help add gloss and sheen and often comes in a quick-dry formula so you don't have to sit around waiting for your polish to dry.

To pick up any excess color that might have gotten on the skin around your nails, take a Q-tip and dip it in some nail polish remover and carefully go around the edges of your nails.

Once your nails are dry, I add a small amount of cuticle oil. This helps hydrate the area, lessening your chances of getting painful hangnails. To answer Carrie's question, I prefer to use cuticle oil because it is more potent than cuticle cream.

To add even more hydration, I like to use a hand cream at night in addition to my cuticle oil. This is especially good to do in the winter when our skin is more dry than normal. One of my favorite hands creams is Jo Malone's Vitamin E Nourishing Hand Treatment.

COLOR, COLOR, COLOR

What nail polish color you decide to use is solely based on your personality. I like to tell people to have fun! If you don't want to push the envelope too much, save the funky colors for your toes and stick to a safer color on your hands. A light pink is always a great choice and is flattering to many different skin tones. Two of my favorites are Essie's Ballet Slippers and Mademoiselle.

Of course, there are always trendy colors like Chanel's Black Satin, Blue Satin, and Vamp, and OPI's Lincoln Park After Dark. I like to wear these on my hands and on my feet. These colors may be too much for some people (like my mom!), so if you're uncomfortable with them on your hands, save them for the pedicure.

A French manicure (natural or pink nail with soft white tips) is always a safe bet and will always be in style, especially for big occasions like weddings. Lots of ladies get a French manicure on their toes, too.

Finally, I could never leave out a ravishing red. There is just something very sexy about red nails. I know most men love a woman with smoking hot red nails, and there's certainly nothing wrong with that!

Straight Buzz

When you store your nail polish, don't keep it in a warm place. The polish will change color and consistency. The refrigerator is a great home for your polish because it will help maintain its smooth consistency.

HOW TO SPEND YOUR BEAUTY BUCKS—MY FAVORITE NAIL PRODUCTS

Some of my favorite nail polish colors from my favorite brands:

Chanel

Black Satin
Khaki Rose
Madness
Paradoxal
Particulière
Rose Satin
Vamp

Deborah Lippmann

Baby Love
Brown Eyed Girl
Hit Me With Your Best Shot
Just Walk Away Renee
P.Y.T.
Sarah Smile
Waking Up in Vegas

Essie

Ballet Slippers
Chinchilly
Hi-Maintenance
Iced Chai Latte

Limo-Scene
Mademoiselle
Sugar Daddy

OPI

I'm Not Really A Waitress
It's A Girl
Lincoln Park After Dark
OPI Red

Hand Creams

Jo Malone Vitamin E Nourishing Hand Treatment
Laura Mercier Hand Cream
La Mer The Hand Treatment
$ Neutrogena Hand Cream Norwegian Formula
   Fragrance Free
$ Nivea Smooth Indulgence Hand Cream

Nail Care Products

Essie Apricot Cuticle Oil
Essie First Base Base Coat
Essie To Dry For
Jessica Nails Brilliance: High Gloss in a Flash
Jessica Nails Fusion
Jessica Nails Nourish Therapeutic Cuticle Formula
Kiehl's Cuticle Cream
OPI Natural Nail Base Coat
OPI Top Coat
Seche Vite Dry Fast Top Coat
SolarOil Cuticle Oil

Star Style

It was never out of the ordinary to have to wait hours (and I do mean plural) to interview Jennifer Lopez. She is a diva through and through and would often make the press wait around to talk to her for what felt like days. My record for her was five hours, and that was for the film *Enough*. Publicists never like to say exactly why their client is running late, but there must have been a back-up publicist working on this particular occasion. Her reason for why we were waiting five hours to interview Jennifer Lopez? Jennifer had to get an "emergency manicure." I had no idea there was such a thing, but wow, five hours? That must have been some manicure!

LIFE-CHANGING LISTS
The Beauty Essentials

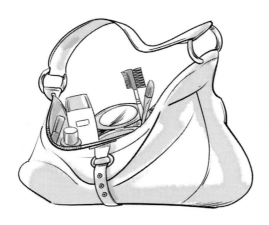

Hopefully, you are now up to speed on all things beauty. But just to make your life even easier (and let's face it, who's going to turn THAT down?), I've put together some quick and easy lists of products and items you need to have with you at all times, as well as ways to make your beauty buying experience even more enjoyable. Are you a "lists" person? I am, because a good list usually cuts to the chase and spells out exactly what you need to know.

So, here it goes—the beauty basics just for you!

TOP FIVE BEAUTY PRODUCTS TO HAVE IN YOUR HANDBAG AT ALL TIMES

1. Lip gloss—if you put nothing else on, at least put on some lip gloss!
2. Pressed powder compact—this is essential to help control shine and for easy touch-ups.
3. Blotting papers—these work wonders to help control oil without causing any disruption to your make-up.
4. Mirror—have a good mirror to make sure everything is in place and looking great.
5. Dental floss—I know I haven't mentioned this at all before, but how many times have you been out to lunch and needed some dental floss in a major way? I always have some with me.

TOP FIVE BEAUTY PRODUCTS THAT MAKE IT LOOK LIKE YOU SPENT TIME ON YOUR MAKE-UP EVEN WHEN YOU HAVEN'T

1. Concealer—this is miracle make-up and can make you look like you've slept eight hours when you've slept just four. Though you might need a cup of coffee to fool yourself!
2. Lip gloss—even if you don't have time for much else, lip gloss gives an instant polish to your face.
3. Powder—another miracle make-up product that can help control shine, even out your complexion, and cover up any blemishes.
4. Mascara—just a quick swipe of mascara on your top lashes will make you look more awake, refreshed, and alive.
5. Eyebrow color—whether you use a pencil or shadow, your brows frame your entire face, so they need to look well-groomed.

TOP FIVE PRODUCTS TO HAVE IN YOUR BEAUTY WARDROBE (A.K.A. THE MEDICINE CABINET)

1. Sunscreen—this needs to be applied every day, 365 days a year, rain or shine.
2. Make-up removers—I use these even before I use my cleanser to make sure I safely remove all of my eye make-up. I also use a cleansing oil on my face.

3. Cleanser—you don't have to spend a lot on a pricey cleanser, but make sure that you do have one that does the job well and removes all that dirt and make-up.

4. Moisturizer—this is essential if you want to keep your skin hydrated and looking fresh and young.

5. Eye cream—also essential to help keep skin hydrated, so lines and wrinkles won't form as quickly.

TOP 5 LIFE-CHANGING BEAUTY BUYS

1. Sunscreen—there is no better beauty product that you can buy than a good-quality sunscreen. It will save your skin and keep you looking younger longer.

2. Eyelash curler—what a huge difference an eyelash curler can make! Your eyes will look bigger instantly.

3. Make-up primer—your make-up will not only stay in place longer, you won't need to do as many make-up touch-ups—which saves you money, since you won't have to replace products as often (except for your mascara—three to four months tops for that one!).

4. Serum—this can penetrate the skin and carry active ingredients beneath the skin's surface, improving tone and texture.

5. Professional eyebrow shaping—even if you only go once, get your brows shaped professionally

so you can see how they are supposed to look.
Then, keep the shape with regular tweezing.

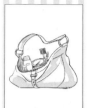

Why am I having all the list-making fun? Take a look in your beauty wardrobe and see what's missing. Write them down, and then flip back through this book and pick some products to test at the beauty counter of your favorite department store. Soon you'll be giving your friends the Straight Buzz on beauty, too!

My Beauty Wardrobe

1. ....

2. ....

3. ....

4. ....

5. ....

Well, that's it for me. I hope you have found all of the tips, tricks, suggestions, and stories in *The Beauty Buzz* helpful. I promised you at the beginning of this book No More Beauty B.S., and, hopefully, you think I delivered the Straight Buzz. Life is too short to get so stressed out about the way you look. Take this book with you the next time you are in the beauty department and feel confident knowing you now have all the answers.

Acknowledgments

There are so many people who made this book possible. I can't thank enough the countless make-up artists and beauty experts who have allowed me to look over their shoulders and ask endless questions while they worked their magic.

A special thank you to my adorable husband, Jeff. Watching him write and market his own book, *Free Publicity*, has been such an inspiration. You are my heart.

Thank you to my sister, Jennifer, whose lipstick application skills would put any make-up artist to shame.

I am lucky to have fantastic friends whose constant encouragement made this book possible—Michelle Lamont, Monica Maynard-Wood, Suzanne Flodin, and Theresa Hernandez.

A big shout-out to all of the amazing MIX 102.9 listeners. I have thoroughly enjoyed answering all of your beauty questions over the years. Without you, this book would never have been written.

Thank you so much to my fantastic co-hosts, Rick O'Bryan and Josh Hart. You both make such an effort to be engaging and enthusiastic during my beauty segments. Thanks for suffering through my endless talk of lipstick and eye shadows.

I must thank the other men in my life, Bob and Dallas. I will need your help next when I write a men's grooming book!

Thanks to my awesome book editor, Erica Lovett. This project was definitely a team effort! And thanks to Milli Brown and the rest of the team at Brown Books.

And a very special thank you to the most beautiful woman in the world, my mother, Dorothy. You have given me the best life possible and all of the tools to write this book. Everything I am I owe to you.

About the Author

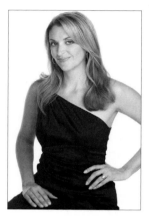

Victoria Snee is an AP award–winning journalist. She has worked in television and radio in Dallas, Texas, since 1996 covering beauty, lifestyle, fashion, and entertainment stories. Victoria regularly interviews major Hollywood stars at award shows, movie premieres, and other red carpet events, picking up beauty secrets from some of the world's most glamorous people. In 2009, she was named one of Dallas' Ten Most Beautiful Women by *D Magazine*. Victoria is a graduate of Southern Methodist University in Dallas with a BA in Broadcast Journalism. She lives in Plano with her husband, Jeff Crilley.

Index